Table of Contents

INTRODUCTION

Mouthwash, mouth rinse or oral rinse is a liquid which is held in the mouth passively or swilled around the mouth by contraction of the perioral muscles and/or movement of the head, and may be gargled, where the head is tilted back and the liquid bubbled at the back of the mouth. Usually mouthwashes are antiseptic solutions intended to reduce the microbial load in the oral cavity, although other mouthwashes might be given for other reasons such as for their analgesic, anti-inflammatory or anti-fungal action. Additionally, some rinses act as saliva substitutes to neutralize acid and keep the mouth moist in xerostomia (dry mouth).

How Mouthwash Works

Mouthwashes or mouth rinses are cosmetic products used to make our mouths feel clean and fresh. They also freshen our breath. They are usually ready-to-use liquids, a liquid concentrate or a powder that is added to water before use. By flushing away small particles of food and germs from teeth, gums and tongue, mouthwashes help to reduce the causes of tooth decay and bad breath. They are not a substitute for brushing our teeth which is the main way of helping prevent tooth decay. However, because mouthwashes reach all parts of the mouth, and areas which cannot be brushed, they can be a useful addition to good mouth hygiene routines.

HOW TO CHOOSE A MOUTHWASH

You have many options, and the right mouthwash or rinse for you is the one that meets your dental hygiene needs for the health of your teeth and gums, and taste preference.

To help choose the right mouthwash or rinse, remember what mouthwash does and keep these points in mind:

• Alcohol - Alcohol is a component of many mouthwashes and rinses, which can problematic if a large quantity is deliberately swallowed. If you want to buy one type of mouthwash or rinse for the whole family, and your household includes school-aged children or teens, you may want to choose from among the alcohol-free mouthwash products that are available. Also, some recovering alcoholics avoid using mouthwash with alcohol in daily oral care because of the potential for abuse.

• Sensitivity - Some people find the ingredients in mouthwash irritating, especially people who have sensitive gums. Also, people who don't usually complain of sensitive gums may find that their mouths are more sensitive for a short time if they are recovering from a dental procedure.If you have a sensitive mouth, consider an alcohol-free or natural mouthwash in your oral care routine. Natural mouthwashes often contain ingredients such as aloe vera and chamomile for a soothing effect.

• Plaque control - If you want a mouthwash that not only helps control bad breath but also helps to prevent plaque build-up on the teeth, look for a dental rinse that contains anti-plaque ingredients. If you're uncertain about which mouthwash or rinse would best meet your oral health needs, ask your dentist or dental hygienist for advice.

TYPES OF MOUTHWASH

There are two main types of mouthwashes:

• Therapeutic mouthwashes. These have active ingredients that kill bacteria and can help reduce plaque, gingivitis, cavities and bad breath. Those that contain fluoride help prevent or reduce tooth decay.

• Cosmetic mouthwashes. These may temporarily control or reduce bad breath and leave your mouth with a pleasant taste, but don't reduce your risk of cavities or gum disease.

Some therapeutic mouthwashes require a prescription, but many mouthwashes are available over-the-counter. Talk to your dentist about whether you need a mouthwash and what kind of mouthwash to use, depending on your dental health needs.

When selecting an over-the-counter mouthwash, look for products that carry the American Dental Association Seal of Acceptance, which means that they have been tested and shown to be safe and effective.

HOW TO USE MOUTHWASH

Using mouthwash correctly can freshen your breath, help prevent cavities and treat gingivitis. There are two main types of mouthwash that you can choose. Cosmetic mouthwash masks bad breath but does not treat the cause of bad breath. Therapeutic mouthwash, on the other hand, does kill the bacteria that causes bad breath while reducing plaque, gingivitis, and cavities. Once you have chosen your mouthwash, use it once a day before or after brushing, or more often if your dentist instructs you to do so.

1. Pour the proper dosage into a small cup. Read the instructions on the label of your mouthwash to learn the proper dosage. Your bottle of mouthwash may have come with a small cup (often the bottle's cap) you can use to measure the correct amount. If your bottle didn't come with a cup, pour the mouthwash into a small cup you've set aside for this specific purpose.

• Most mouthwashes will recommend a dose of about 20 ml.[8] This amount is enough to clean your teeth in one dose. Some fluoride mouthwashes, however, only require 10 ml.

• Unless you're using a prescription mouthwash, don't worry too much about using the exact amount. Use enough mouthwash to fill your mouth without making you feel uncomfortable. Always follow your dentist's instructions when using a prescription mouthwash.

2. Pour it into your mouth. Tip the cup into your mouth and pour in all of the mouthwash at once. Close your mouth to create a seal so that the mouthwash won't squirt out when you start swishing it. Do not swallow the mouthwash. It may contain strong chemicals that are not meant to be ingested.

3. Swish it through your teeth for 30 seconds to a minute. Follow the directions on the bottle to learn exactly how long you should swish the mouthwash. Make sure it swishes in front of and behind your teeth. Swish it through your molars as well as your front teeth. Swish it under your tongue and across the roof of your mouth, too.

4. Spit it out. When you're done swishing, spit it out into the sink. Rinse out the sink to get rid of the used mouthwash.

5. It is not a replacement: It is essential to remember that no mouthwash is a replacement for the regular oral care routine of twice-daily brushing and daily flossing. So, even if your dentist recommends or prescribes a mouthwash, you still need to follow your complete oral care routine to maintain good dental health. The main function of most mouthwashes is to freshen breath, although if you suffer from severe chronic bad breath (halitosis), talk to your dentist about other ways to address the causes of the problem and manage your condition.

Depending on what type of mouthwash you used, you might need to wait 1/2 hour or more before drinking water or eating in order to increase the effectiveness of the mouthwash. Read the directions on the bottle to find out if you should wait.

WHEN TO USE MOUTHWASH

1. Use it before or after brushing. According to the American Dental Association, it doesn't matter whether you use mouthwash before or after brushing - both are equally effective. The more important thing is to use good quality mouthwash.

2. Use it to freshen your breath anytime. You can carry a little bottle of mouthwash with you during the day to refresh your breath after meals. If you have a problem with bad breath, this can be a good alternative to popping breath mints all day long.

3. Don't substitute it for brushing and flossing. Mouthwash is meant to be a supplement to other oral hygiene practices - not a replacement. Make sure you continue to brush and floss your teeth as recommended by your dentist. In most cases you should brush twice a day and floss once. Use mouthwash every time you brush, or just in the morning or at night - it's your choice.

4. Ask your dentist for more information. If you're using mouthwash in an attempt to treat gingivitis, chronic bad breath, or cavities, you should make an appointment with your dentist to make sure you're using the right mouthwash. Mouthwash alone may not be effective enough to treat the problem you're dealing with, so it's important to get dental care before things get worse.

WHY USE MOUTHWASH

There are several reasons to make mouthwash part of your oral hygiene routine.

Mouthwash can help get your teeth cleaner and whiter. Using a mouthwash or rinse can help prevent or reduce tartar, plaque, and gingivitis (early-stage gum disease). Some mouth rinses also contain ingredients to help whiten teeth.

Mouthwash complements brushing and flossing. Mouthwashes and rinses can help remove any plaque that may still be left after brushing and flossing. They can also help rinse food particles out of the mouth.

Mouthwash can help tame bad breath. Bad breath can have many different causes.

Improper oral hygiene: Proper tooth and tongue brushing and flossing can make all the difference if you suffer from bad breath. Without proper oral hygiene, food particles and bacteria left in the mouth after eating can cause bad breath. It is important to learn the proper way to brush and floss. Along with brushing and flossing, you can use mouthwashes and rinses to kill the bacteria that can cause bad breath. This helps leave your mouth with a fresher smell.

• **Food**: Foods such as garlic and onions are especially known to contribute to bad breath. When we eat, the food is absorbed into the bloodstream and transferred to our lungs. As we breathe the odour is expelled, causing bad breath. This lasts until our body has eliminated the food. If you cannot properly brush or floss your teeth immediately after eating, try to rinse your mouth with water – this will help to dislodge food particles and moisten your mouth. If your meal comes with raw parsley as a garnish, chew on it – it's a natural breath freshener!

• **Smoking**: Along with the damage that smoking does to our overall health, teeth, and gums, it is also a cause of bad breath.

• **Medications**: Some drugs, such as antihistamines and decongestants, cause bad breath by making your mouth dry. Dry mouth, which is explained next, is a contributor to bad breath.

• **Dry mouth (xerostomia):** Dry mouth occurs when the flow of saliva decreases. As previously mentioned, it can be a side effect of certain medications. Dry mouth can also be caused by salivary gland problems, excessive talking, exercising, dieting, smoking, continuous breathing through the mouth or drinking alcohol. To prevent and treat dry mouth it is helpful to drink lots of water or to use sugarless candy or gum. This will stimulate saliva flow that will then cleanse the mouth and remove particles and bacteria that cause odour.

• **Gum disease (periodontal disease):** Periodontal disease is a bacterial infection of the gums that support the teeth. Individuals who suffer from gum disease are more prone to bad breath as it creates the perfect breeding ground for odour-causing bacteria to flourish. Normally the tiny space in between your gums and teeth is 1 mm to 3 mm. When you have periodontal disease the space (periodontal pockets) can grow to 5 mm or more. This allows bacteria to hide in deeper and more secluded areas.

• **Other medical disorders**: Medical disorders that can cause bad breath include respiratory infections, chronic sinusitis, chronic bronchitis, postnasal drip, diabetes, and gastrointestinal, liver, or kidney problems.

If you have persistent bad breath that has not been treatable by proper oral hygiene techniques, you should consult with your dentist. Bad breath can often be a warning sign of periodontal disease or respiratory infection.

BENEFITS OF USING MOUTHWASH

Mouthwash is an effective tool in the fight against tooth decay, gingivitis, as well as the promotion of healthy teeth and gums. Here are just a couple benefits from using mouthwash.

1)   Freshens breath – First and foremost, and most obviously, mouthwash temporarily reduces bad breath. With a variety of flavours to choose from, mouthwash kills bacteria associated with causing bad breath leaving you with minty fresh breath.

2)   Prevents Plaque build-up – Various mouthwashes help prevent plaque build up on your gums, in-between teeth, and on the surface of your teeth in between brushing. Although it prevents the build up of plague, it cannot reduce the plaque that already exists on your teeth. So remember to always brush and floss to remove the plaque before it becomes a problem.

3)   Removes particles – Most people use mouthwash only after brushing. While this is a good practice, mouthwash can also be used before brushing to rinse out any loose particles in your mouth making your brushing and flossing more effective.

4)   Stop cavities from forming – With regular use of mouthwash before and after you brush and floss, you can

reduce the chances of cavities forming. Mouthwashes that contain fluoride can prevent cavities and strengthen your enamel. Remember, not all mouthwashes contain fluoride. Be sure to check the label on your mouthwash before purchasing.

Studies have shown that oral rinses can reduce more plaque and more signs of gingivitis when used in addition to tooth brushing compared with tooth brushing alone. Whatever oral rinse you choose, be sure to follow the instructions and avoid swallowing.

With regular brushing, flossing, and the use of mouthwash you can keep your mouth healthy and smelling fresh. Talk with your dentist about the importance of mouthwash and find a strategy that works for you.

RISKS OF USING MOUTHWASH

1. Oral cancer and dry mouth

Alcohol-based mouthwashes are the kind that you find in most grocery stores but they can have some serious side effects. The alcohol itself can dry out your mouth and lead to bad breath which is likely what you're trying to avoid by using a mouthwash to begin with. There is an ongoing debate about whether alcohol-based mouthwashes increase your risk for oral cancer. This is still being researched and a recent systematic review and meta-analysis failed to find an association between alcohol-based mouthwash use and oral cancer but the jury is still out on this.

2. It could raise your blood pressure

There are studies that have indicated that regular use of mouthwash could increase your blood pressure because it eliminates some of the beneficial bacteria found in the mouth. Not all bacteria is bad bacteria and mouthwash can eliminate the bacteria responsible for producing nitric oxide that helps in protecting your cardiovascular system.

3. It can eliminate good bacteria

When you wipe out all of the bacteria in your mouth, you wipe out your first line of protection against invading bacteria. For this reason, using mouthwash can increase your risk of getting infections like H Pylori and C-difficile. Antibacterial mouthwash can increase your risk of gut inflammation that can lead to increased intestinal permeability and contribute to food intolerances, food allergies, and even some gut-related autoimmune diseases.

Whether you choose to use a mouthwash or not, you should know that mouthwash of any kind is not recommended for children younger than 6 years of age. The swallowing reflexes of children this young may not be well developed and that can result in them swallowing large amounts of mouthwash which can trigger nausea, vomiting, and intoxication (due to the alcohol content in some mouthwashes).

When shopping for a mouthwash, consider what the most important benefits of mouthwash are for you. Look for alcohol-free options so that you don't have to worry about the risks associated with an alcohol-based mouthwash. Be sure to look for an ADA approved mouthwash and check to make sure it addresses the issues you're looking to treat. If you find yourself unsure, don't hesitate to ask your dentist for help.

MOUTHWASH INGREDIENTS

• Alcohol: Alcohol is added to mouthwash not to destroy bacteria but to act as a carrier agent for essential active ingredients such as menthol, eucalyptol and thymol which help to penetrate plaque. Sometimes a significant amount of alcohol (up to 27% vol) is added, as a carrier for the flavor, to provide "bite" Because of the alcohol content, it is possible to fail a breathalyzer test after rinsing although breath alcohol levels return to normal after 10 minutes. In addition, alcohol is a drying agent, which encourages bacterial activity in the mouth, releasing more malodorous volatile sulfur compounds. Therefore, alcohol-containing mouthwash may temporarily worsen halitosis in those who already have it, or indeed be the sole cause of halitosis in other individuals.

• Benzydamine/Difflam (analgesics): In painful oral conditions such as aphthous stomatitis, analgesic mouthrinses (e.g. benzydamine mouthwash, or Difflam) are sometimes used to ease pain, commonly used before meals to reduce discomfort while eating.

• Betamethasone: Betamethasone is sometimes used as an anti-inflammatory, corticosteroid mouthwash. It may be used for severe inflammatory conditions of the oral mucosa such as the severe forms of aphthous stomatitis.

• Cetylpyridinium chloride (antiseptic, antimalodor): Cetylpyridinium chloride containing mouthwash is used in some specialized mouthwashes for halitosis. Cetylpyridinium chloride mouthwash has less anti-plaque effect than chlorhexidine and may cause staining of teeth, or sometimes an oral burning sensation or ulceration.

• Chlorhexidine digluconate and Hexetidine (antiseptic): Chlorhexidine digluconate is a chemical antiseptic and is used in a 0.12–0.2% solution as a mouthwash. However, there is no evidence to support that higher concentrations are more effective in controlling dental plaque and gingivitis. It has anti-plaque action, but also some anti-fungal action. It is especially effective against Gram-negative rods. The proportion of Gram-negative rods increase as gingivitis develops so it is also used to reduce gingivitis. It is sometimes used as an adjunct to prevent dental caries and to treat gingivitis periodontal disease.

• Essential oils and phenols: Phenolic compounds include essential oil constituents that have some antibacterial properties, like phenol, thymol, eugenol or eucalyptol. Essential oils are oils which have been extracted from plants. Mouthwashes based on essential oils could be more effective than traditional mouthcare - for anti-gingival treatments.

• Fluoride (anticavity): Anti-cavity mouth rinses use fluoride to protect against tooth decay. Most people using fluoridated toothpastes do not require fluoride-containing mouth rinses, rather fluoride mouthwashes are sometimes used in individuals who are at high risk of dental decay.

• Tetracycline (antibiotic): Tetracycline is an antibiotic which may sometimes be used as a mouthwash in adults (it causes red staining of teeth in children). It is sometimes use for herpetiforme ulceration (an uncommon type of aphthous stomatitis), but prolonged use may lead to oral candidiasis as the fungal population of the mouth overgrows in the absence of enough competing bacteria.

ADVANTAGES OF MOUTHWASH

• Cut down on cavities. It is absolutely true that rinsing with a fluoride rinse can help reduce cavities. There are countless studies on the benefits of fluoride in reducing demineralization and cavitations of the teeth.

• Fight gum disease. With periodontal disease (such as gingivitis), gums and tooth sockets can get inflamed or infected because of plaque from bacteria and food that lingers on teeth. An antibacterial mouthwash, like one with alcohol or chlorhexidine, may help prevent periodontal disease.

• Soothe canker sores. Mouthwash can ease a canker sore by detoxing the area — reducing the amount of bacteria that can irritate the site. In many cases, a simple saltwater rinse will do.

• Safeguard your pregnancy. Periodontal disease is actually a risk factor for giving birth to preterm, low-weight babies — the bacteria from a gum infection can get into a pregnant woman's bloodstream and increase inflammatory markers, which in turn can stimulate contractions. And a recent study published in the American Journal of Obstetrics and Gynecology (which received funding from Proctor and Gamble) found that moms-to-be who used mouthwash throughout their pregnancy were less likely to go into early labor.

Mouthwash clearly offers certain benefits but, it is important to know that not all mouth rinses are the same. Saltwater rinses can be made at home with warm water and salt, whereas store-bought types contain a variety of ingredients ranging from fluoride (Act) to alcohol (Listerine) to chlorhexidine (Peridex).

DISADVANTAGES OF MOUTHWASH

Mouthwash is by no means a cure-all. In fact, mouthwash gets bad marks because it:

• Irritates canker sores. If the alcohol content of your mouth rinse is too high, it may actually end up irritating the canker sore more than helping it.

• Masks bad breath. "Mouthwash can lead to fresher breath, but it may be short-lived. If a patient has poor oral hygiene and doesn't brush effectively, there is no amount of mouthwash that can mask the effects of poor health. Just using mouthwash would be equivalent to not bathing and using cologne to mask the smell.

• Soreness, ulceration and redness may sometimes occur (e.g. aphthous stomatitis, allergic contact stomatitis) if the person is allergic or sensitive to mouthwash ingredients such as preservatives, coloring, flavors and fragrances.

TIPS FOR USING MOUTHWASH

You're already a pro at brushing and flossing, but you may have some questions about the proper use of mouthwash. You may be wondering whether mouthwash should be used before or after brushing. The American Dental Association explains that manufacturers may recommend a certain order to maximize the product's effectiveness, so you should check the label of your chosen mouthwash. In cases where the manufacturer doesn't make a recommendation, you can rinse either before or after you brush, depending on your preference.

The ideal frequency of mouthwash use is another question you may have. Tufts School of Dental Medicine explains that this depends on the reason you're using the mouthwash. For people who simply want to keep their teeth clean, Tufts recommends swishing with mouthwash twice per day. For people who want the benefits of fluoride, once per day is enough.

While mouthwash can be a good addition to an oral hygiene routine, it's not a replacement for proper brushing and flossing. Make sure to keep brushing twice per day and flossing once per day, even when you're using mouthwash.

Choosing the right mouthwash doesn't have to be complicated. When you go to the store, keep your main oral health concerns in mind and select a product that meets those specific needs.

RECIPES

Baking Soda

What You Will Need

• ½ teaspoon of baking soda or sodium bicarbonate

• ½ glass of warm water

What You Have To Do

• Add half a teaspoon of table salt to half a glass of warm water.

• Mix well and rinse your mouth after or before brushing your teeth.

How Often You Should Do This –

• You can do this 3-4 times daily.

Why This Works

• Baking soda is a great fix for bad breath and oral bacteria. Its alkaline nature can increase salivary pH. This can help neutralize the acids produced by oral bacteria upon consumption of soda drinks and caffeine.

Coconut Oil

What You Will Need

• 1 tablespoon of virgin coconut oil

What You Have To Do

• Swish a tablespoon of virgin coconut oil in your mouth for 10-15 minutes.

• Spit the oil and go about your oral care routine.

How Often You Should Do This

• You must do this once daily, prior to brushing your teeth.

Why This Works

• Oil pulling with coconut oil is not only good for your oral hygiene but is also a great way to detoxify your body. It can help in decreasing plaque formation as well as plaque-induced gingivitis.

Peppermint Oil

What You Will Need

• 2-3 drops of peppermint essential oil

• 1 cup of distilled water

What You Have To Do

• Add two to three drops of peppermint oil to a cup of distilled water.

• Mix well and use this solution to rinse your mouth.

How Often You Should Do This

• You may do this 2-3 times daily, preferably after every meal.

Why This Works

• Peppermint oil mouthwashes are especially effective in combating halitosis (bad breath).

Cinnamon Oil

What You Will Need

• 2-3 drops of cinnamon essential oil

• 1 cup of distilled water

What You Have To Do

• Add two to three drops of cinnamon essential oil to a cup of distilled water.

• Mix well.

• Use this mixture to rinse your mouth.

How Often You Should Do This

• You may do this multiple times daily.

Why This Works

• Cinnamon oil is antibacterial and is effective in the treatment of dental caries caused by oral bacteria.

Tea Tree Oil

What You Will Need

• 1-2 drops of tea tree oil

• ½ cup of distilled water

What You Have To Do

• Add one to two drops of tea tree oil to half a cup of distilled water.

• Mix well and use the mixture to rinse your mouth.

How Often You Should Do This

• You may do this 2-3 times daily, preferably after every meal.

Why This Works

• The anti-inflammatory nature of this essential oil can be quite beneficial in reducing the symptoms of bleeding and inflammation triggered by gingivitis.

Salt

What You Will Need

• ½ teaspoon of table salt

• ½ glass of warm water

What You Have To Do

• Add half a teaspoon of table salt to half a glass of warm water.

• Mix well and rinse your mouth using the mixture.

How Often You Should Do This

• You can do this 2-3 times daily, following a meal.

Why This Works

• Rinsing your mouth with salt water is almost as effective as any other over-the-counter mouthwashes that contain compounds like chlorhexidine. It can help in reducing dental plaque as well as the oral microbial count.

Aloe Vera Juice

What You Will Need

• ½ cup of aloe vera juice

• ½ cup of distilled water

• ½ teaspoon of baking soda

What You Have To Do

• Mix half a cup of aloe vera juice with half a cup of distilled water.

• Rinse your mouth using this mixture after brushing your teeth.

How Often You Should Do This

• You can do this 3-4 times daily.

Why This Works

• Aloe vera mouth rinses can be effective in reducing periodontal indices. They can also help reduce gingival bleeding and plaque.

Clove

What You Will Need

- 1/4 cup vodka or 1/4 cup gin

- 1/2 cup distilled water

- 1/4 teaspoon honey

- 1/4 teaspoon ground cinnamon

- 1/2 teaspoon clove oil

What You Have To Do

• Mix everything together and stir until the honey is dissolved.

• Pour 4 tsps. in a glass and rinse your mouth for 30 seconds.

How Often You Should Do This

• You can do this 3-4 times daily.

Why This Works

• Clove oil fights dental pain, toothaches, sore gums and mouth ulcers very effectively.

All these recipes are great alternatives to the vast number of over-the-counter mouthwashes. With these recipes in hand, you don't have to worry about your oral rinses running out! They can be prepared in a jiffy, that too, while sitting in the comfort of your home.

NATURAL MOUTHWASHES

In order to avoid possible toxins like thymol, which is known to be dangerous to the environment as well as to aquatic organisms, and hexetidine, considered to be carcinogenic, you might also save some of your hard-earned cash and even see better results by making your own mouthwash.

Super Citrus Oil Mouthwash

Ingredients:

• 2 cups of filtered water

• 2 teaspoons of calcium carbonate powder

• 1 teaspoon of xylitol crystals

• 10 drops of trace mineral liquid

• 10 drops of peppermint essential oil

• 5 drops of lemon essential oil

• 3 drops of wild orange essential oil

Instructions:

In a mason jar, or other similar container with a lid, stir together the xylitol crystals and the calcium powder. Add the essential oils and liquid minerals. Stir again to be sure everything is well combined. Add your water and stir. Close the lid and shake for 1 minute. That's it! How easy was that?! You can find all these ingredients in your local natural or health food store or online. Store this in the refrigerator (it keeps for 2 to 3 weeks) and shake well before each use.

Xylitol is a natural sweetener proven to have a positive effect on tooth and gum health. It is recommended by many dentists and is now a popular ingredient in natural toothpaste, gum and mouthwash. It will also improve the taste and even the effectiveness of your mouthwash.

Super Simple Mouthwash

Ingredients:

• 1 cup of filtered water

• 4 teaspoons of baking soda

• 4 drops of tea tree essential oil

• 4 drops of peppermint essential oil

Instructions:

Add all ingredients to a mason jar or similar container with a lid. Shake very well. Use about 2 tablespoons of this mixture each day, the same way you would use mouthwash for super white teeth and fresh breath. The baking soda will usually settle to the bottom of the container after a few hours, but don't worry, this is normal. Simply shake well before each use.

Cinnamon and Honey Mouthwash

Ingredients:

• 2 organic lemons, juiced

• ½ tablespoon of cinnamon powder

• 1 teaspoon of baking soda (not baking powder!)

• 5 teaspoons of raw, organic honey

• 1 cup of warm water

Instructions:

Using a mason jar or similar type of container with a tight fitting lid, add all ingredients in the order given. Be sure the water is very warm as it needs to melt the honey. Close the lid and shake for one minute. Store in the fridge and use two tablespoons as a mouth rinse.

Three-Ingredient Mouthwash

Ingredients:

- 1 cup of filtered water

- 1 teaspoon of baking soda

- 3 drops of peppermint essential oil

Instructions:

Add all ingredients in a glass jar with a tight-fitting lid and shake very well. This can be kept in the bathroom and does not require refrigeration. Shake well before each use.

Grandma's Disinfecting Mouthwash

Ingredients:

- 1 cup of filtered water

- 2 tablespoons of apple cider vinegar

Instructions:

Mix the ingredients together in a glass jar with a tight-fitting lid. Shake well before each use. This will keep forever right on your bathroom countertop.

Herb-Infused Mouthwash

Ingredients:

• 2 cups of filtered water

• ½ ounce of whole cloves

• 1 ounce of Oregon grape root

• 1 ounce of rosemary sprigs

Instructions:

Boil the water and then add all remaining ingredients to the water. Boil for one minute, then turn off the fire and cover the pot. Allow herbs to steep in the water overnight. Strain out the herbs with a piece of cheesecloth in the morning and store in a glass container with a tight-fitting lid. Shake well before each use and store in the refrigerator. This will keep 7 to 14 days in the fridge.

Simple Hydrogen Peroxide Whitening Mouthwash

Ingredients:

• 1-part filtered water1-part hydrogen peroxide

• 1 tablespoon of water

Instructions:

Don't make a large batch of this solution. Try one tablespoon of hydrogen peroxide and one tablespoon of water, for example. Mix in a ceramic or glass container (such as a glass or coffee cup) and use immediately. Swish in the mouth for 30 seconds and then spit it out. Do not swallow, and do not save any extra solution.

Sweet-Smelling Essential Oil Mouthwash

Ingredients:

• 1 cup of filtered water

• 20 drops of the essential oil of your choice. Best choices are cinnamon, clove, wintergreen, peppermint, or tea tree oil

Instructions:

In a glass container with a tight fitting lid, combine all ingredients and shake well. Always shake well before each use. This mixture will keep on the kitchen counter or bathroom counter forever.

Since ancient times, turmeric has been used for remedying oral ailments, among other therapeutic applications too numerous to count. Studies have shown that using turmeric as part of a mouth cleansing solution can be more effective than a chemical mouthwash. The curcumin in turmeric acts to disrupt the cycle of dental plaque formation. Research has found that turmeric extract and turmeric oil may reverse precancerous changes in oral submucous fibrosis in humans and even kill oral cancer cells.

REASONS TO USE A NATURAL MOUTHWASH

Using a natural mouthwash in conjunction with regular brushing and flossing is a good way to reduce oral bacteria and maintain (or achieve) optimal oral health and hygiene. Also known as a mouth rinse, oral rinse or tonic, a natural alcohol-free mouthwash may be the right choice for you.

Here are great reasons:

Natural mouthwash uses time-tested ingredients. Shop for Dental Herb Company products online.

• In a market dominated by the use of synthetic additives, many of the long-term health effects of these relatively new substances such as sodium lauryl sulfate (SLS) and triclosan are still unknown. A natural mouth rinse, such as Dental Herb Company's Tooth & Gums Tonic, uses pure essential oils (distilled liquids extracted from flowers, leaves, bark, stems, roots, shrubs and trees) and botanicals – ingredients that have been known for their medicinal benefits for thousands of years. Three of the most commonly used essential oils in natural mouthwash and other natural mouth care products are peppermint, cinnamon and lavender. Research has proven the efficacy of their antibacterial, antimicrobial, and anti-inflammatory properties.

Natural mouthwash is gentle for even the most sensitive mouths.

• Medical conditions, medications, and even brushing habits can cause oral sensitivity. When the mouth is particularly susceptible, choosing gentler options such as natural toothpaste and alcohol-free mouthwash can prevent further discomfort. Botanical extracts condition oral tissue and offer hydration to help soothe sensitive oral tissue.

Natural mouthwash feels great.

• Most commercial mouth rinses contain alcohol to kill bacteria, and anyone who has used an alcohol-based mouthwash is familiar with their burning sensation. While alcohol is effective on a short-term basis, the eventual result is that our bodies develop a resistance to the antibiotics found in these mouth care products. Furthermore, their burning discomfort can be unpleasant enough for consumers to want to discontinue this part of their oral care routine. Using a mouthwash can help decrease the risk of gingivitis and gum disease. An alcohol-free mouth rinse is better because it is equally effective at eradicating germs without the irritation.

Natural mouthwash has naturally antibacterial properties.

• The antibacterial effect of essential oils in a natural mouth rinse has been shown to be highly effective in preventing gum disease without contributing to the rise of antibacterial-resistant bacteria. Many commercial mouthwashes use the additive Triclosan as an antibacterial agent. Although effective in preventing gum disease, studies have raised some concerns about its potential for making bacteria resistant to antibiotics.

Natural mouthwash contains no harsh additives.

• Alcohol, triclosan and sodium lauryl sulfate (SLS) can be harsh on oral tissue—particularly for those with compromised immune functioning. Diabetics, patients undergoing chemotherapy, and those with rheumatoid arthritis are more prone to developing gum disease and experiencing oral irritation from synthetic ingredients.Using a non alcoholic mouthwash and toothpaste can prevent uncomfortable and unnecessary side effects.

Natural mouthwash is effective.

• The essential oils and herbal extracts found in a natural mouth rinse such as Dental Herb Company's Tooth & Gums Tonic are valued for their therapeutic properties. Natural preservative free oral rinses that contain certain essential oils offer antibacterial, anti-inflammatory, antimicrobial and antifungal properties typically not found in most commercial mouth wash products.

Natural mouthwash doesn't cause dry mouth.

• Dry mouth (xerostomia) can be a side effect of certain medications, chemotherapy or lifestyle choices. Regular use of an alcohol-based mouth rinse can also result in a decreased production of saliva. Dry mouth is as potentially detrimental to oral health as it is uncomfortable, and insufficient saliva increases the risk for cavities and gum disease. You can reduce your risk by choosing a natural alcohol free mouth rinse.

Natural mouthwash helps keep your mouth (and body) healthy

• Oral health is an excellent indicator of overall health. Infections of the oral mucosa can result in inflammation in other parts of the body because the oral mucosa provides a direct pathway into the bloodstream. Use a natural mouth rinse and toothpaste for highly effective cleansing and to help protect against gum disease.

Natural mouthwash contains no "mystery" ingredients.

• Reading ingredient labels is not only daunting, it can be confusing. If you don't like the idea of not recognizing (or being able to pronounce) the ingredients in your products, then choosing natural oral care products is the right choice for you.

CONCLUSION

When used properly, mouthwash can make contributions to oral health, but the product is not a cure-all of dental problems. Dental dentists and science proves that brushing and flossing daily are the best behaviors for effectively reducing plaque. Combining those efforts with regular dental exams and cleanings from a screened dentist is the best way to effectively reducing harmful plaque.